The Best Dash Recipes For Your Health

The Everyday Guide For Your Delicious Breakfast

Candace Hickman

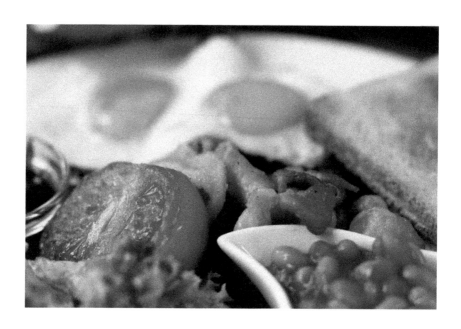

TABLE OF CONTENT

Cinnamon Plums 7

Apples Bowls.. 9

Strawberry Oats 11

Almond Peach Mix 12

Dates Rice 14

Pomegranate Yogurt...................................... 16

Coconut Porridge 17

Berries Rice 18

Coconut Rice 20

Vanilla Rice and Cherries 22

Rice Bowls.. 24

Hash Browns Casserole.................................. 26

Mushroom and Rice Mix................................. 28

Tomato Eggs 30

Scallions Omelet.. 33

Zucchini Almond Oatmeal............................... 35

Maple Almonds Bowl 37

Mint Chickpeas Salad 38

Millet Pudding 41

Lemon Chia Bowls 43

Cinnamon Tapioca Pudding............................. 45

Coconut Hash 46

Carrot and Peas Salad 48

Chia Oats 50

Almond Scones... 52

Almond Cookies 54

Cinnamon Oats 56

Banana Muffins 58

Almond Pancakes.. 61

Berries Pancakes 63

Cashew Parfait... 65

Almond Potato Waffles 67

Coconut Toast 70

Coconut Cocoa Oats 72

Cherries Oatmeal 76

Pecan Bowls.. 78

Baked Peaches 79

Apple Oats 81

Pomegranate Oats 83

Carrots Hash 86

Spring Omelet 88

Cheese Frittata.. 90

Eggs and Artichokes 92

Beans Bake 94

Mozzarella Scramble 97

Cheddar Hash Browns 99

Chives Risotto *101*

Coconut Quinoa *104*

Cherries Bowls...*106*

Cinnamon Plums

Preparation time: 10 minutes

Cooking time: 15 minutes

Servings: 4

Ingredients:

- 4 plums, pitted and halved
- 3 tablespoons coconut oil, melted
- ½ teaspoon cinnamon powder
- 1 cup coconut cream
- ¼ cup unsweetened coconut, shredded
- 2 tablespoons sunflower seeds, toasted

Directions:

1. In a baking dish, combine the plums with the oil, cinnamon and the other ingredients, introduce in the oven and bake at 380 degrees F for 15 minutes.
2. Divide everything into bowls and serve.

Nutrition info per serving: 282 calories, 2.3g protein, 12.4g carbohydrates, 27.1g fat, 2.8g fiber, 0mg cholesterol, 10mg sodium, 289mg potassium

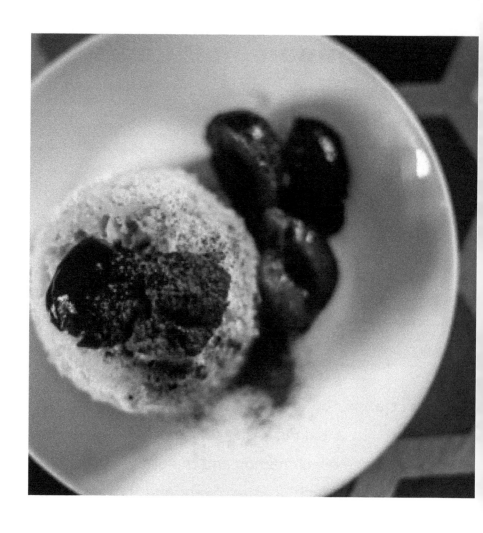

Apples Bowls

Preparation time: 10 minutes

Cooking time: 0 minutes

Servings: 4

Ingredients:

- 6 apples, cored and pureed
- 1 cup natural apple juice
- 2 tablespoons coconut sugar
- 2 cups non-fat yogurt
- 1 teaspoon cinnamon powder

Directions:

1. In a bowl, combine the apples with the apple juice and the other ingredients, stir, divide into bowls and keep in the fridge for 10 minutes before serving.

Nutrition info per serving: 279 calories, 4.4g protein, 69.5g carbohydrates, 0.6g fat, 8.9g fiber, 3mg cholesterol, 56mg sodium, 379mg potassium

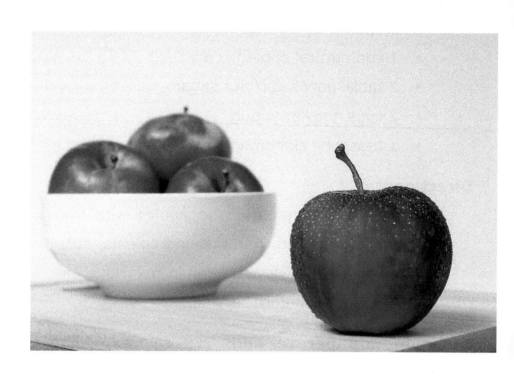

Strawberry Oats

Preparation time: 10 minutes

Cooking time: 20 minutes

Servings: 4

Ingredients:

- 1 and ½ cups gluten-free oats
- 2 and ¼ cups almond milk
- ½ teaspoon vanilla extract
- 2 cups strawberries, sliced
- 2 tablespoons coconut sugar

Directions:

1. Put the milk in a pot, bring to a simmer over medium heat, add the oats and the other ingredients, stir, cook for 20 minutes, divide into bowls and serve for breakfast.

Nutrition info per serving: 226 calories, 6.4g protein, 42.5g carbohydrates, 3.6g fat, 8.4g fiber, 0mg cholesterol, 46mg sodium, 158mg potassium

Almond Peach Mix

Preparation time: 10 minutes

Cooking time: 15 minutes

Servings: 4

Ingredients:

- 4 peaches, cored and cut into wedges
- ¼ cup maple syrup
- ¼ teaspoon almond extract
- ½ cup almond milk

Directions:

1. Put the almond milk in a pot, bring to a simmer over medium heat, add the peaches and the other ingredients, toss, cook for 15 minutes, divide into bowls and serve for breakfast.

Nutrition info per serving: 180 calories, 2.1g protein, 28.9g carbohydrates, 7.6g fat, 3g fiber, 0mg cholesterol, 6mg sodium, 404mg potassium

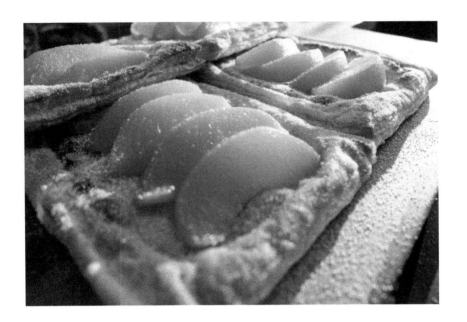

Dates Rice

Preparation time: 10 minutes

Cooking time: 20 minutes

Servings: 4

Ingredients:

- 1 cup brown rice
- 2 cups almond milk
- 4 dates, chopped
- 2 tablespoons cinnamon powder
- 2 tablespoons coconut sugar

Directions:

1. In a pot, combine the rice with the milk and the other ingredients, bring to a simmer and cook over medium heat for 20 minutes.
2. Stir the mix again, divide into bowls and serve for breakfast.

Nutrition info per serving: 231 calories, 3.8g protein, 51.2g carbohydrates, 1g fat, 1.5g fiber, 0mg cholesterol, 40mg sodium, 108mg potassium

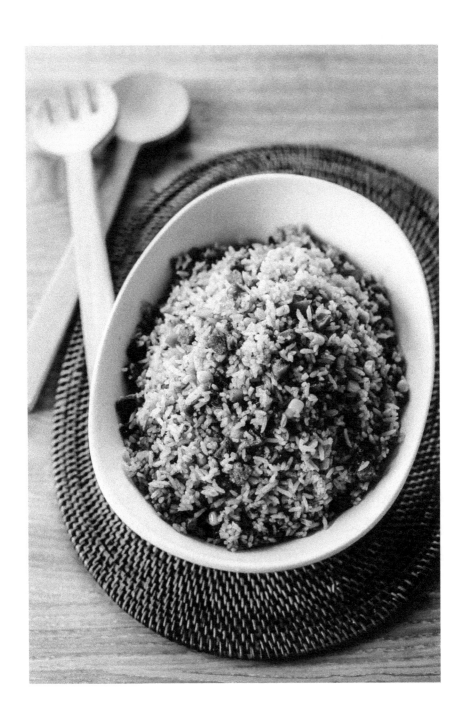

Pomegranate Yogurt

Preparation time: 10 minutes

Cooking time: 0 minutes

Servings: 4

Ingredients:

- 1 cup figs, halved
- 1 pear, cored and cubed
- ½ cup pomegranate seeds
- ½ cup coconut sugar
- 2 cups non-fat yogurt

Directions:

1. In a bowl, combine the figs with the yogurt and the other ingredients, toss, divide into bowls and serve for breakfast.

Nutrition info per serving: 315 calories, 8.9g protein, 73.5g carbohydrates, 0.7g fat, 6.1g fiber, 2mg cholesterol, 100mg sodium, 691mg potassium

Coconut Porridge

Preparation time: 10 minutes

Cooking time: 20 minutes

Servings: 4

Ingredients:

- 4 cups coconut milk
- 1 cup cornmeal
- 1 teaspoon vanilla extract
- 1 cup strawberries, halved
- ½ teaspoon nutmeg, ground

Directions:

1. Put the milk in a pot, bring to a simmer over medium heat, add the cornmeal and the other ingredients, toss, cook for 20 minutes, and take off the heat.
2. Divide the porridge between plates and serve for breakfast.

Nutrition info per serving: 678 calories, 8.2g protein, 39.8g carbohydrates, 58.5g fat, 8.3g fiber, 0mg cholesterol, 47mg sodium, 776mg potassium

Berries Rice

Preparation time: 10 minutes

Cooking time: 20 minutes

Servings: 4

Ingredients:

- 1 cup brown rice
- 2 cups coconut milk
- 1 tablespoon cinnamon powder
- 1 cup blackberries
- ½ cup coconut cream, unsweetened

Directions:

1. Put the milk in a pot, bring to a simmer over medium heat, add the rice and the other ingredients, cook for 20 minutes, and divide into bowls.
2. Serve warm for breakfast.

Nutrition info per serving: 463 calories, 6.8g protein, 46.3g carbohydrates, 30.1g fat, 6.2g fiber, 0mg cholesterol, 20mg sodium, 501mg potassium

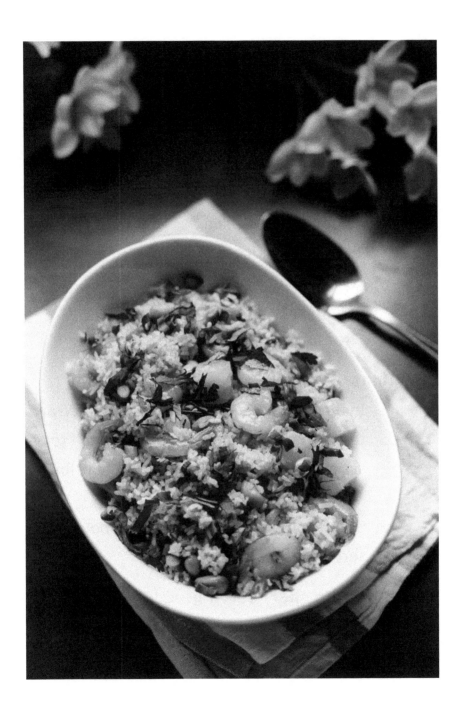

Coconut Rice

Preparation time: 10 minutes

Cooking time: 20 minutes

Servings: 6

Ingredients:

- 2 cups coconut milk
- 1 cup brown rice
- 2 tablespoons coconut sugar
- ¾ cup coconut cream
- 1 teaspoon vanilla extract

Directions:

1. In a pot, combine the milk with the rice and the other ingredients, stir, bring to a simmer and cook over medium heat for 20 minutes.
2. Stir the mix again, divide into bowls and serve for breakfast.

Nutrition info per serving: 317 calories, 4g protein, 34.2g carbohydrates, 19.3g fat, 2.2g fiber, 0mg cholesterol, 25mg sodium, 247mg potassium

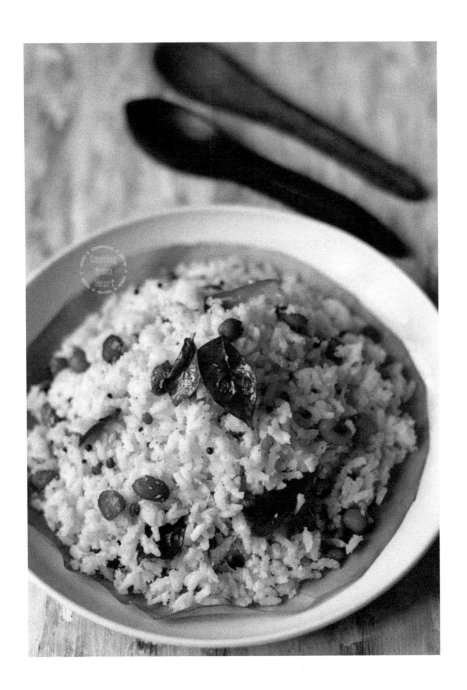

21

Vanilla Rice and Cherries

Preparation time: 10 minutes

Cooking time: 25 minutes

Servings: 4

Ingredients:

- 1 tablespoon coconut, shredded
- 2 tablespoons coconut sugar
- 1 cup brown rice
- 2 cups coconut milk
- ½ teaspoon vanilla extract
- ¼ cup cherries, pitted and halved
- Cooking spray

Directions:

1. Put the milk in a pot, add the sugar and the coconut, stir and bring to a simmer over medium heat.
2. Add the rice and the other ingredients, simmer for 25 minutes stirring often, divide into bowls and serve.

Nutrition info per serving: 484 calories, 6.1g protein, 52.7g carbohydrates, 29.3g fat, 3.4g fiber, 0mg cholesterol, 38mg sodium, 379mg potassium

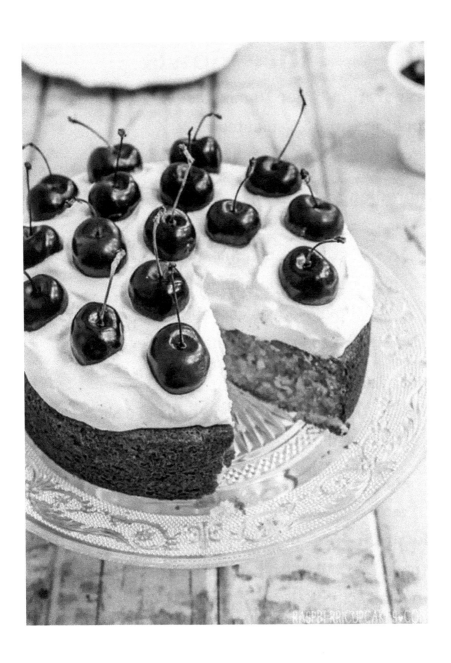

Rice Bowls

Preparation time: 10 minutes

Cooking time: 25 minutes

Servings: 4

Ingredients:

- 1 cup brown rice
- 2 cups almond milk
- 1 tablespoon ginger, grated
- 3 tablespoons coconut sugar
- 1 teaspoon cinnamon powder

Directions:

1. Put the milk in a pot, bring to a simmer over medium heat, add the rice and the other ingredients, stir, cook for 25 minutes, divide into bowls and serve.

Nutrition info per serving: 483 calories, 6.2g protein, 53.6g carbohydrates, 29g fat, 3.4g fiber, 0mg cholesterol, 21mg sodium, 387mg potassium

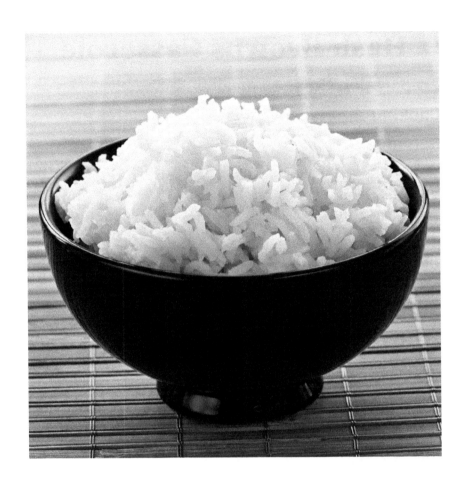

Hash Browns Casserole

Preparation time: 10 minutes

Cooking time: 35 minutes

Servings: 4

Ingredients:

- 1 pound hash browns
- 4 eggs, whisked
- 1 red onion, chopped
- 1 chili pepper, chopped
- 1 tablespoon olive oil
- 6 ounces low-sodium sausage, chopped
- ¼ teaspoon chili powder
- A pinch of black pepper

Directions:

1. Heat up a pan with the oil over medium heat, add the onion and the sausage, stir and brown for 5 minutes.
2. Add the hash browns and the other ingredients except the eggs and pepper, stir and cook for 5 minutes more.
3. Pour the eggs mixed with the black pepper over the sausage mix, introduce the pan in

the oven and bake at 370 degrees F for 25 minutes.

4. Divide the mix between plates and serve for breakfast,

Nutrition info per serving: 357 calories, 15.2g protein, 19.4g carbohydrates, 24.8g fat, 1.7g fiber, 204mg cholesterol, 241mg sodium, 522mg potassium

Mushroom and Rice Mix

Preparation time: 10 minutes

Cooking time: 30 minutes

Servings: 4

Ingredients:

- 1 red onion, chopped
- 1 cup brown rice
- 2 garlic cloves, minced
- 2 tablespoons olive oil
- 2 cups low-sodium chicken stock
- 1 tablespoon cilantro, chopped
- ½ cup fat-free cheddar cheese, grated
- ½ pound white mushroom, sliced
- Black pepper to the taste

Directions:

1. Heat up a pan with the oil over medium heat, add the onion, garlic and mushrooms, stir and cook for 5-6 minutes.
2. Add the rice and the rest of the ingredients, bring to a simmer and cook over medium heat for 25 minutes stirring often.

3. Divide the rice mix between bowls and serve for breakfast.

Nutrition info per serving: 314 calories, 9.5g protein, 42.1g carbohydrates, 12.2g fat, 1.8g fiber, 15mg cholesterol, 162mg sodium, 295mg potassium

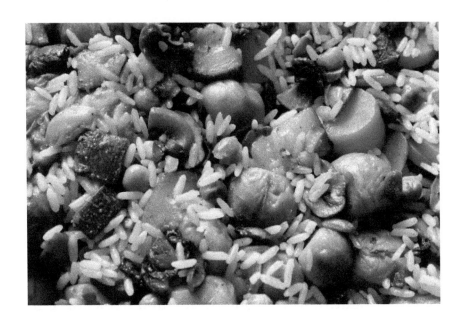

Tomato Eggs

Preparation time: 10 minutes

Cooking time: 20 minutes

Servings: 4

Ingredients:

- ½ cup low-fat milk
- Black pepper to the taste
- 8 eggs, whisked
- 1 cup baby spinach, chopped
- 1 yellow onion, chopped
- 1 tablespoon olive oil
- 1 cup cherry tomatoes, cubed
- ¼ cup fat-free cheddar, grated

Directions:

1. Heat up a pan with the oil over medium heat, add the onion, stir and cook for 2-3 minutes.
2. Add the spinach and tomatoes, stir and cook for 2 minutes more.
3. Add the eggs mixed with the milk and black pepper and toss gently.

4. Sprinkle the cheddar on top, introduce the pan in the oven and cook at 390 degrees F for 15 minutes.
5. Divide between plates and serve.

Nutrition info per serving: 201 calories, 15.3g protein, 7g carbohydrates, 12.7g fat, 1.3g fiber, 330mg cholesterol, 216mg sodium, 352mg potassium

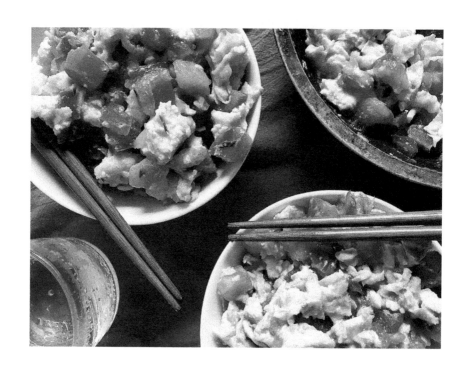

Scallions Omelet

Preparation time: 5 minutes

Cooking time: 15 minutes

Servings: 4

Ingredients:

- 4 eggs, whisked
- A pinch of black pepper
- 1 tablespoon olive oil
- 1 teaspoon sesame seeds
- 2 scallions, chopped
- 1 teaspoon sweet paprika
- 1 tablespoon cilantro, chopped

Directions:

1. Heat up a pan with the oil over medium heat, add the scallions, stir and sauté for 2 minutes.
2. Add the eggs mixed with the other ingredients, toss a bit, spread the omelet into the pan and cook for 7 minutes.
3. Flip, cook the omelet for 6 minutes more, divide between plates and serve.

Nutrition info per serving: 101 calories, 5.9g protein, 1.4g carbohydrates, 8.3g fat, 0.5g fiber, 164mg cholesterol, 63mg sodium, 97mg potassium

Zucchini Almond Oatmeal

Preparation time: 5 minutes

Cooking time: 20 minutes

Servings: 4

Ingredients:

- 1 cup steel cut oats
- 3 cups almond milk
- 1 tablespoon fat-free butter
- 2 teaspoons cinnamon powder
- 1 teaspoon pumpkin pie spice
- 1 cup zucchinis, grated

Directions:

1. Heat up a pan with the milk over medium heat, add the oats and the other ingredients, toss, bring to a simmer and cook for 20 minutes, stirring from time to time.
2. Divide the oatmeal into bowls and serve for breakfast.

Nutrition info per serving: 508 calories, 7.5g protein, 27.2g carbohydrates, 44.5g fat, 6.7g fiber, 0mg cholesterol, 63mg sodium, 624mg potassium

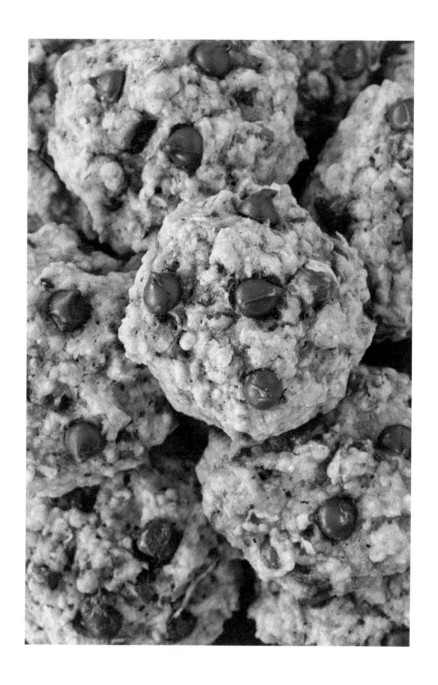

Maple Almonds Bowl

Preparation time: 5 minutes

Cooking time: 20 minutes

Servings: 4

Ingredients:

- 2 cups coconut milk
- 1 cup coconut, shredded
- ½ cup maple syrup
- 1 cup raisins
- 1 cup almonds
- ½ teaspoon vanilla extract

Directions:

1. Put the milk in a pot, bring to a simmer over medium heat, add the coconut and the other ingredients, and cook for 20 minutes, stirring from time to time.
2. Divide the mix into bowls and serve warm for breakfast.

Nutrition info per serving: 697 calories, 9g .6protein, 70g carbohydrates, 47.4g fat, 8.8g fiber, 0mg cholesterol, 30mg sodium, 914mg potassium

Mint Chickpeas Salad

Preparation time: 5 minutes

Cooking time: 15 minutes

Servings: 4

Ingredients:

- 2 garlic cloves, minced
- 2 tomatoes, roughly cubed
- 1 cucumber, roughly cubed
- 2 shallots, chopped
- 2 cups canned chickpeas, no-salt-added, drained
- 1 tablespoon parsley, chopped
- 1/3 cup mint, chopped
- 1 avocado, pitted, peeled and diced
- 2 tablespoons olive oil
- Juice of 1 lime
- Black pepper to the taste

Directions:

1. Heat up a pan with the oil over medium heat, add the garlic and the shallots, stir and cook for 2 minutes.

2. Add the chickpeas and the other ingredients, toss, cook for 13 minutes more, divide into bowls and serve for breakfast.

Nutrition info per serving: 563 calories, 21.9g protein, 73g carbohydrates, 23.1g fat, 22.5g fiber, 0mg cholesterol, 36mg sodium, 1455mg potassium

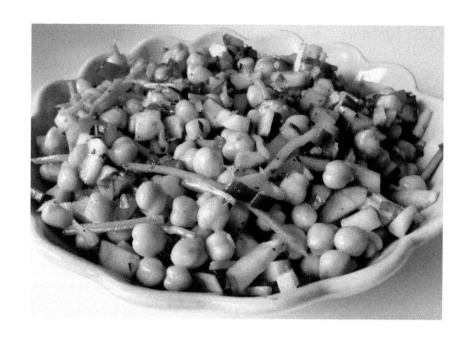

Millet Pudding

Preparation time: 10 minutes

Cooking time: 30 minutes

Servings: 4

Ingredients:

- 14 ounces coconut milk
- 1 cup millet
- 1 tablespoon cocoa powder
- ½ teaspoon vanilla extract

Directions:

1. Put the milk in a pot, bring to a simmer over medium heat, add the millet and the other ingredients, and cook for 30 minutes stirring often.
2. Divide into bowls and serve for breakfast.

Nutrition info per serving: 422 calories, 8g protein, 42.7g carbohydrates, 25.9g fat, 6.8g fiber, 0mg cholesterol, 18mg sodium, 393mg potassium

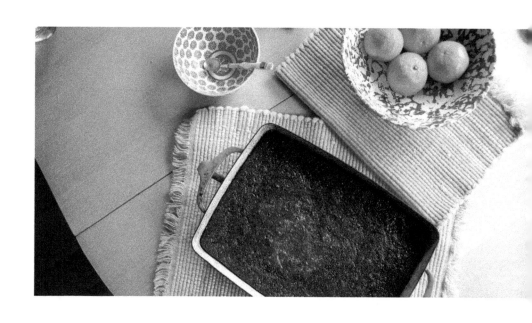

Lemon Chia Bowls

Preparation time: 15 minutes

Cooking time: 0 minutes

Servings: 4

Ingredients:

- 2 cups almond milk
- ½ cup chia seeds
- 2 tablespoons coconut sugar
- Zest of ½ lemon, grated
- 1 teaspoon vanilla extract
- ½ teaspoon ginger powder

Directions:

1. In a bowl, combine the chia seeds with the milk and the other ingredients, toss and leave aside for 15 minutes before serving.

Nutrition info per serving: 375 calories, 52.g protein, 19.5g carbohydrates, 33g fat, 7.7g fiber, 0mg cholesterol, 21mg sodium, 387mg potassium

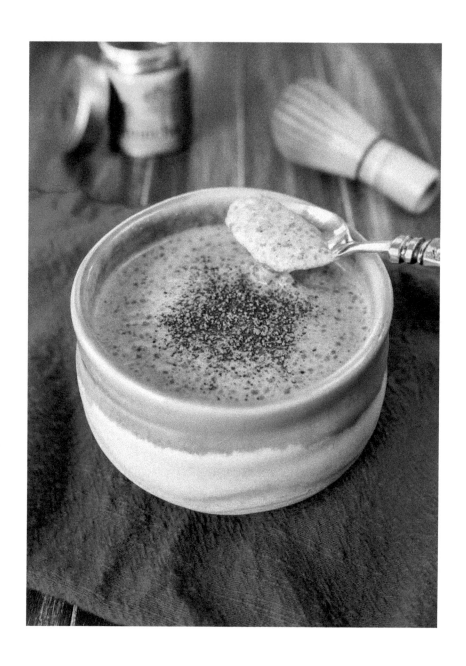

Cinnamon Tapioca Pudding

Preparation time: 2 hours

Cooking time: 0 minutes

Servings: 4

Ingredients:

- ½ cup tapioca pearls
- 2 cups coconut milk, hot
- 4 teaspoons coconut sugar
- ½ teaspoon cinnamon powder

Directions:

1. In a bowl, combine the tapioca with the hot milk and the other ingredients, stir and leave aside for 2 hours before serving.
2. Divide into small bowls and serve for breakfast.

Nutrition info per serving: 359 calories, 2.8g protein, 27.5g carbohydrates, 28.6g fat, 2.8g fiber, 0mg cholesterol, 18mg sodium, 318mg potassium

Coconut Hash

Preparation time: 10 minutes

Cooking time: 25 minutes

Servings: 4

Ingredients:

- 1 pound hash browns, low sodium
- 1 tablespoon avocado oil
- 1/3 cup coconut cream
- 1 yellow onion, chopped
- 1 cup fat-free cheddar cheese, grated
- Black pepper to the taste
- 4 eggs, whisked

Directions:

1. Heat up a pan with the oil over medium heat, add the hash browns and the onion, stir and sauté for 5 minutes.
2. Add the rest of the ingredients except the cheese, toss and cook for 5 minutes more.
3. Sprinkle the cheese on top, introduce the pan in the oven and cook at 390 degrees F for 15 minutes.

4. Divide the mix between plates and serve for breakfast.

Nutrition info per serving: 238 calories, 18.1g protein, 11g carbohydrates, 13.4g fat, 1.2g fiber, 170mg cholesterol, 518mg sodium, 163mg potassium

Carrot and Peas Salad

Preparation time: 10 minutes

Cooking time: 20 minutes

Servings: 4

Ingredients:

- 3 garlic cloves, minced
- 1 yellow onion, chopped
- 1 tablespoon olive oil
- 1 carrot, chopped
- 1 tablespoon balsamic vinegar
- 2 cups snow peas, halved
- ½ cup veggie stock, no-salt-added
- 2 tablespoons scallions, chopped
- 1 tablespoon cilantro, chopped

Directions:

1. Heat up a pan with the oil over medium heat, add the onion and the garlic, stir and cook for 5 minutes.
2. Add the snow peas and the other ingredients, toss and cook over medium heat for 15 minutes.

3. Divide the mix into bowls and serve warm
   for breakfast.

Nutrition info per serving: 89 calories, 3.4g
protein, 11.2g carbohydrates, 3.7g fat, 3.5g fiber,
0mg cholesterol, 33mg sodium, 318mg potassium

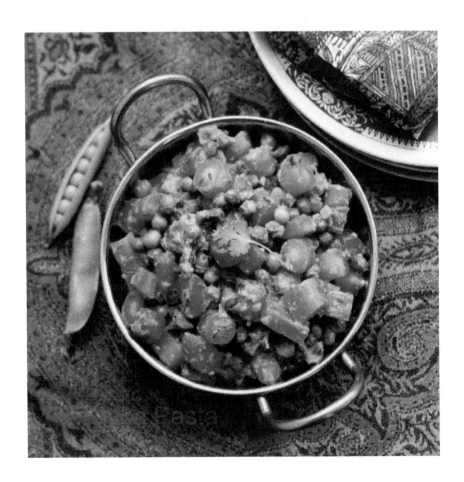

Chia Oats

Preparation time: 6 hours and 10 minutes

Cooking time: 0 minutes

Servings: 1

Ingredients:

- 1 tablespoon chia seeds
- ½ cup almond milk
- 2 tablespoons natural peanut butter
- 1 tablespoon stevia
- ½ cup gluten-free oats
- 2 tablespoons raspberries

Directions:

1. In a mason jar, combine the oats with the chia seeds and the other ingredients except the raspberries, stir a bit, cover and keep in the fridge for 6 hours.
2. Top with the raspberries and serve for breakfast.

per serving: 628 calories, 17.8g protein, 34g carbohydrates, 50.3g fat, 12g fiber, 0mg cholesterol, 31mg sodium, 396mg potassium.

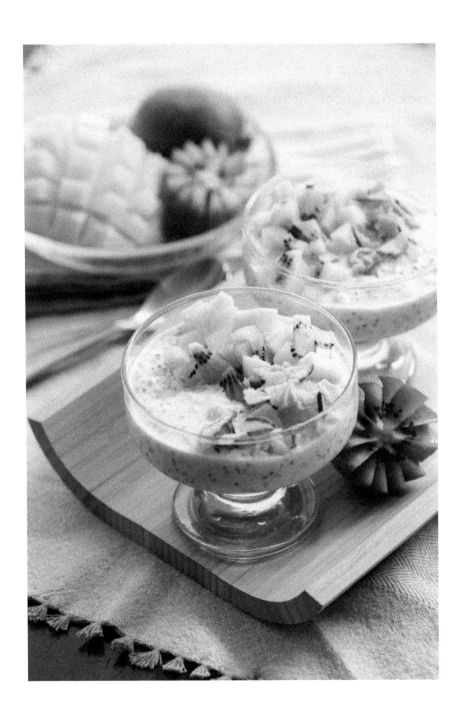

Almond Scones

Preparation time: 10 minutes

Cooking time: 12 minutes

Servings: 8

Ingredients:

- 2 cups almond flour
- ½ teaspoon baking soda
- ¼ cup cranberries, dried
- ¼ cup sunflower seeds
- ¼ cup apricots, chopped
- ¼ cup walnuts, chopped
- ¼ cup sesame seeds
- 2 tablespoons stevia
- 1 egg, whisked

Directions:

1. In a bowl, combine the flour with the baking soda, cranberries, and the other ingredients and stir well.
2. Shape a square dough, roll onto a floured working surface and cut into 16 squares.

3. Arrange the squares on a baking sheet lined with parchment paper and bake the scones at 350 degrees F for 12 minutes.
4. Serve the scones for breakfast.

Nutrition info per serving: 110 calories, 4.3g protein, 4.1g carbohydrates, 9.4g fat, 1.9g fiber, 20mg cholesterol, 90mg sodium, 77mg potassium.

Almond Cookies

Preparation time: 10 minutes

Cooking time: 15 minutes

Servings: 12

Ingredients:

- 1 cup almond butter
- ¼ cup stevia
- 1 teaspoon vanilla extract
- 2 bananas, peeled and mashed
- 2 cups gluten-free oats
- 1 teaspoon cinnamon powder
- 1 cup almonds, chopped
- ½ cup raisins

Directions:

1. In a bowl, combine the butter with the stevia and the other ingredients and stir well using a hand mixer.
2. Scoop medium molds of this mix on a baking sheet lined with parchment paper and flatten them a bit.
3. Cook them at 325 degrees F for 15 minutes and serve for breakfast.

Nutrition info per serving: 166 calories, 4.9g protein, 24.8g carbohydrates, 6.3g fat, 4.9g fiber, 0mg cholesterol, 1mg sodium, 184mg potassium

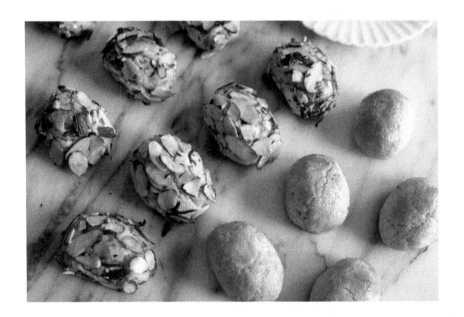

Cinnamon Oats

Preparation time: 10 minutes

Cooking time: 7 hours

Servings: 5

Ingredients:

- 2 apples, cored, peeled and cubed
- 1 cup gluten-free oats
- 1 and ½ cups of water
- 1 and ½ cups of almond milk
- 2 tablespoons swerve
- 2 tablespoons almond butter
- ½ teaspoon cinnamon powder
- 1 tablespoon flax seed, ground
- Cooking spray

Directions:

1. Grease a slow cooker with the cooking spray and combine the oats with the water and the other ingredients inside.
2. Toss a bit and cook on Low for 7 hours.
3. Divide into bowls and serve for breakfast.

Nutrition info per serving: 201 calories, 5.2g protein, 38.5g carbohydrates, 6.8g fat, 6.8g fiber, 0mg cholesterol, 44mg sodium, 155mg potassium

Banana Muffins

Preparation time: 10 minutes

Cooking time: 25 minutes

Servings: 12

Ingredients:

- 2 bananas, peeled and mashed
- 1 cup almond milk
- 1 teaspoon vanilla extract
- ¼ cup pure maple syrup
- 1 teaspoon apple cider vinegar
- ¼ cup coconut oil, melted
- 2 cups almond flour
- 4 tablespoons coconut sugar
- 2 teaspoons cinnamon powder
- 2 teaspoons baking powder
- 2 cups blueberries
- ½ teaspoon baking soda
- ½ cup walnuts, chopped

Directions:

1. In a bowl, combine the bananas with the almond milk, vanilla, and the other ingredients and whisk well.

58

2. Divide the mix into 12 muffin tins and bake at 350 degrees F for 25 minutes.
3. Serve the muffins for breakfast.

Nutrition info per serving: 209 calories, 3.1g protein, 19.5g carbohydrates, 14.9g fat, 2.4g fiber, 0mg cholesterol, 59mg sodium, 267mg potassium

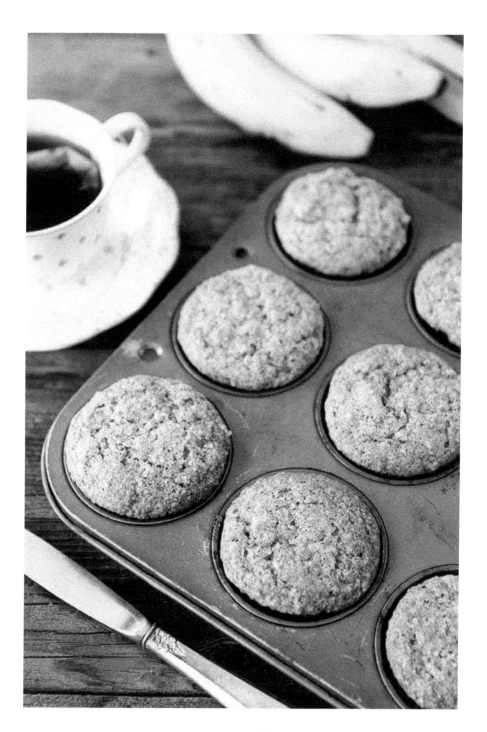

Almond Pancakes

Preparation time: 10 minutes

Cooking time: 6 minutes

Servings: 12

Ingredients:

- 1 cup almond flour
- 1 tablespoon flaxseed, ground
- 2 cups of coconut milk
- 2 tablespoons coconut oil, melted
- 1 teaspoon cinnamon powder
- 2 teaspoons stevia

Directions:

1. In a bowl, combine the flour with the flaxseed, milk, half of the oil, cinnamon, and stevia and whisk well.

2. Heat a pan with the rest of the oil over medium heat, add ¼ cup of the crepes batter, spread into the pan, cook for 2-3 minutes on each side and transfer to a plate.

3. Repeat with the rest of the crepes batter and serve them for breakfast.

Nutrition info per serving: 128 calories, 1.5g protein, 2.9g carbohydrates, 13.2g fat, 1.3g fiber, 0mg cholesterol, 7mg sodium, 110mg potassium

Berries Pancakes

Preparation time: 10 minutes

Cooking time: 7 minutes

Servings: 12

Ingredients:

- 2 eggs, whisked
- 4 tablespoons almond milk
- 1 cup full-fat yogurt
- 3 tablespoons coconut butter, melted
- ½ teaspoon vanilla extract
- 1 and ½ cups almond flour
- 2 tablespoons stevia
- 1 cup blueberries
- 1 tablespoon avocado oil

Directions:

1. In a bowl, combine the eggs with the almond milk and the other ingredients except the oil and whisk well.
2. Heat a pan with the oil over medium heat, add ¼ cup of the batter, spread into the pan, cook for 4 minutes, flip, cook for 3 minutes more and transfer to a plate.

3. Repeat with the rest of the batter and serve the pancakes for breakfast.

Nutrition info per serving: 82 calories, 2.6g protein, 5.1g carbohydrates, 6.1g fat, 1.5g fiber, 28mg cholesterol, 20mg sodium, 57mg potassium

Cashew Parfait

Preparation time: 10 minutes

Cooking time: 0 minutes

Servings: 4

Ingredients:

- ¼ cup cashews
- ½ cup of water
- 2 teaspoons pumpkin pie spice
- 2 cups pumpkin puree
- 2 tablespoons maple syrup
- 1 pear, cored, peeled and chopped
- 2 cups of coconut yogurt

Directions:

1. In a blender, combine the cashews with the water and the other ingredients except the yogurt and pulse well.
2. Divide the yogurt into bowls, also divide the pumpkin cream on top and serve.

Nutrition info per serving: 200 calories, 5.5g protein, 32.9g carbohydrates, 6.4g fat, 5.1g fiber, 0mg cholesterol, 10mg sodium, 367mg potassium

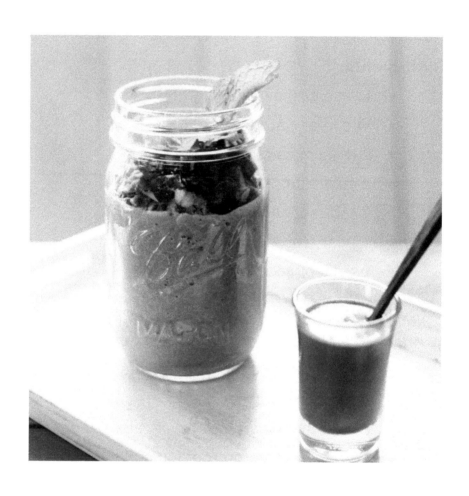

Almond Potato Waffles

Preparation time: 10 minutes

Cooking time: 10 minutes

Servings: 6

Ingredients:

- ½ cup sweet potato, cooked, peeled and grated
- 1 cup almond milk
- 1 cup gluten-free oats
- 2 eggs, whisked
- 1 tablespoon honey
- ¼ teaspoon baking powder
- 1 tablespoon olive oil
- Cooking spray

Directions:

1. In a bowl, combine the sweet potato with the almond milk and the rest of the ingredients except the cooking spray and whisk well.
2. Grease the waffle iron with the cooking spray and pour 1/3 of the batter in each mold.

3. Cook the waffles for 3-4 minutes and serve them for breakfast.

Nutrition info per serving: 234 calories, 5.6g protein, 22.3g carbohydrates, 14.9g fat, 5.1g fiber, 55mg cholesterol, 33mg sodium, 227mg potassium

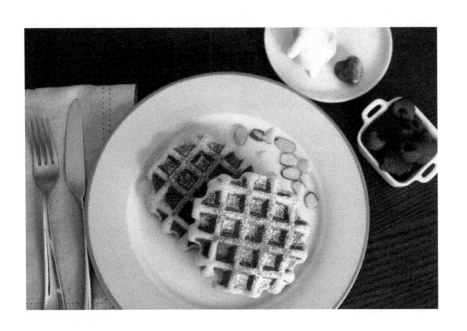

Coconut Toast

Preparation time: 10 minutes

Cooking time: 5 minutes

Servings: 2

Ingredients:

- 4 whole-wheat bread slices
- 2 tablespoons coconut sugar
- ½ cup of coconut milk
- 2 eggs, whisked
- 1 teaspoon vanilla extract
- Cooking spray

Directions:

1. In a bowl, combine the sugar with the milk, eggs, and the vanilla and whisk well.
2. Dip each bread slice in this mix.
3. Heat a pan greased with cooking spray over medium heat, add the French toast, cook for 2-3 minutes on each side, divide between plates and serve for breakfast.

Nutrition info per serving: 390 calories, 14.2g protein, 39.1g carbohydrates, 20.6g fat, 5.1g fiber, 164mg cholesterol, 335mg sodium, 359mg potassium

Coconut Cocoa Oats

Preparation time: 10 minutes

Cooking time: 20 minutes

Servings: 4

Ingredients:

- 2 cups almond milk
- 1 cup old-fashioned oats
- 2 tablespoons coconut sugar
- 1 teaspoon cocoa powder
- 2 teaspoons vanilla extract

Directions:

1. Heat up a pot with the milk over medium heat, add the oats and the other ingredients, bring to a simmer and cook for 20 minutes.
2. Divide the oats into bowls and serve warm for breakfast.

Nutrition info per serving: 381 calories, 5.5g protein, 26.7g carbohydrates, 30g fat, 4.8g fiber, 0mg cholesterol, 19mg sodium, 403mg potassium

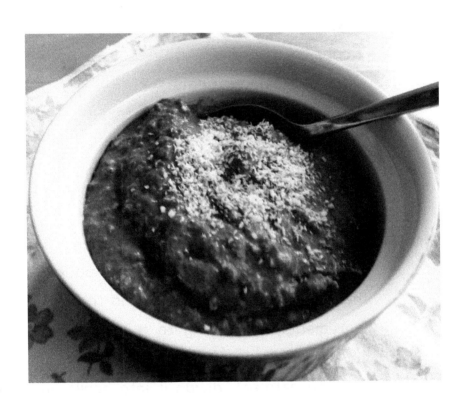

Mango Oats

Preparation time: 10 minutes

Cooking time: 20 minutes

Servings: 4

Ingredients:

- 2 cups coconut milk
- 1 cup old-fashioned oats
- 1 cup mango, peeled and cubed
- 3 tablespoons almond butter
- 2 tablespoons coconut sugar
- ½ teaspoon vanilla extract

Directions:

1. Put the milk in a pot, heat it up over medium heat, add the oats and the other ingredients, stir, bring to a simmer and cook for 20 minutes.
2. Stir the oatmeal, divide it into bowls and serve.

Nutrition info per serving: 473 calories, 8.3g protein, 34.7g carbohydrates, 36.8g fat, 6.5g fiber, 0mg cholesterol, 20mg sodium, 548mg potassium

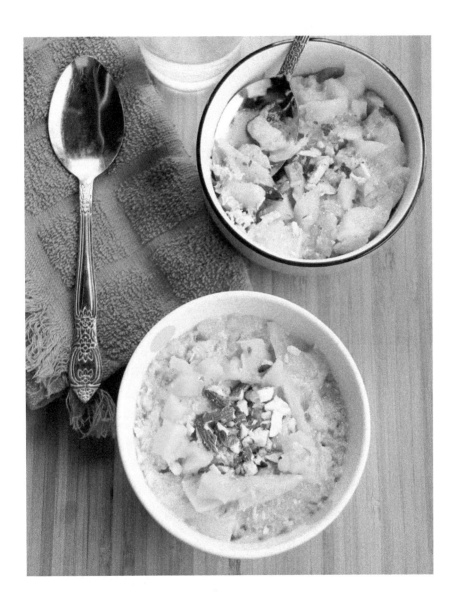

Cherries Oatmeal

Preparation time: 10 minutes

Cooking time: 10 minutes

Servings: 6

Ingredients:

- 2 cups old-fashioned oats
- 3 cups almond milk
- 2 and ½ tablespoons cocoa powder
- 1 teaspoon vanilla extract
- 10 ounces cherries, pitted
- 2 pears, cored, peeled and cubed

Directions:

1. In your pressure cooker, combine the oats with the milk and the other ingredients, toss, cover and cook on High for 10 minutes.
2. Release the pressure naturally for 10 minutes, stir the oatmeal one more time, divide it into bowls and serve.

Nutrition info per serving: 483 calories, 7.5g protein, 51.1g carbohydrates, 31.1g fat, 9.1g fiber, 0mg cholesterol, 30mg sodium, 657mg potassium

Pecan Bowls

Preparation time: 10 minutes

Cooking time: 20 minutes

Servings: 4

Ingredients:

- 1 cup steel cut oats
- 2 cups orange juice
- 2 tablespoons coconut butter, melted
- 2 tablespoons stevia
- 3 tablespoons pecans, chopped
- ¼ teaspoon vanilla extract

Directions:

1. Heat up a pot with the orange juice over medium heat, add the oats, the butter and the other ingredients, whisk, simmer for 20 minutes, divide into bowls and serve for breakfast.

Nutrition info per serving: 238 calories, 4.8g protein, 29.8g carbohydrates, 11.8g fat, 4.6g fiber, 0mg cholesterol, 2mg sodium, 351mg potassium

Baked Peaches

Preparation time: 10 minutes

Cooking time: 20 minutes

Servings: 4

Ingredients:

- 2 cups coconut cream
- 1 teaspoon cinnamon powder
- 1/3 cup palm sugar
- 4 peaches, stones removed and cut into wedges
- Cooking spray

Directions:

1. Grease a baking pan with the cooking spray and combine the peaches with the other ingredients inside.
2. Bake this at 360 degrees F for 20 minutes, divide into bowls and serve for breakfast.

Nutrition info per serving: 395 calories, 4.2g protein, 36.7g carbohydrates, 29g fat, 4.6g fiber, 4.9mg cholesterol, 54mg sodium, 601mg potassium

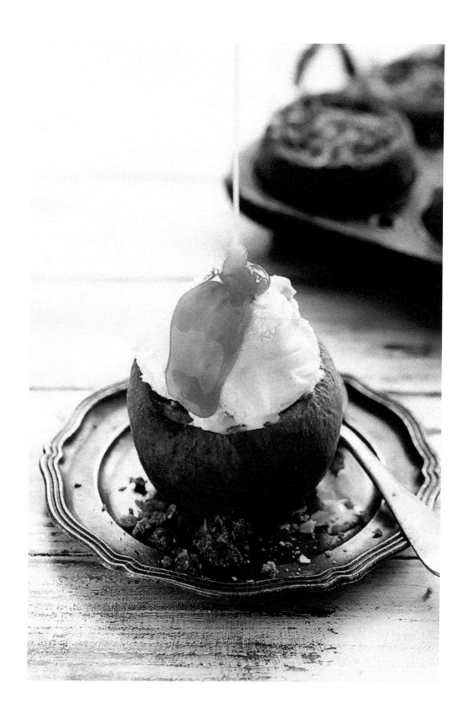

Apple Oats

Preparation time: 10 minutes

Cooking time: 15 minutes

Servings: 4

Ingredients:

- 1 cup steel cut oats
- 1 and ½ cups almond milk
- 1 cup non-fat yogurt
- ¼ cup maple syrup
- 2 apples, cored, peeled and chopped
- ½ teaspoon cinnamon powder

Directions:

1. In a pot, combine the oats with the m ilk and the other ingredients except the yogurt, toss, bring to a simmer and cook over medium-high heat for 15 minutes.
2. Divide the yogurt into bowls, divide the apples and oats mix on top and serve for breakfast.

Nutrition info per serving: 303 calories, 6g protein, 64g carbohydrates, 3.3g fat, 4.8g fiber, 3mg cholesterol, 161mg sodium, 234mg potassiu

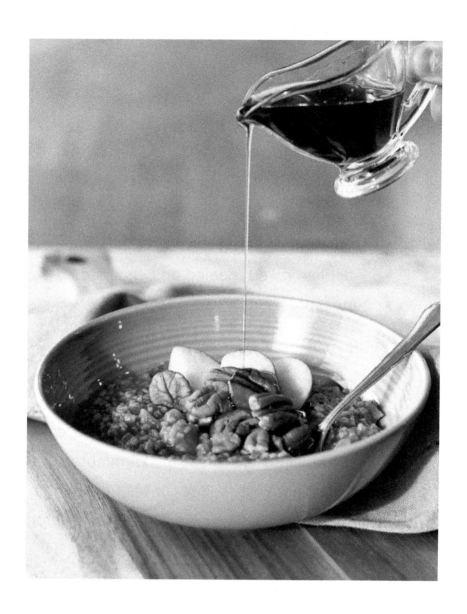

Pomegranate Oats

Preparation time: 10 minutes

Cooking time: 20 minutes

Servings: 4

Ingredients:

- 3 cups almond milk
- 1 cup steel cut oats
- 1 tablespoon cinnamon powder
- 1 mango, peeled, and cubed
- ½ teaspoon vanilla extract
- 3 tablespoons pomegranate seeds

Directions:

1. Put the milk in a pot and heat it up over medium heat.
2. Add the oats, cinnamon and the other ingredients, toss, simmer for 20 minutes, divide into bowls and serve for breakfast.

Nutrition info per serving: 546 calories, 7.5g protein, 37.1g carbohydrates, 44.6g fat, 7.4g fiber, 0mg cholesterol, 29mg sodium, 689mg potassium

Chia Bowls

Preparation time: 10 minutes

Cooking time: 20 minutes

Servings: 4

Ingredients:

- ½ cup steel cut oats
- 2 cups almond milk
- ¼ cup pomegranate seeds
- 4 tablespoons chia seeds
- 1 teaspoon vanilla extract

Directions:

1. Put the milk in a pot, bring to a simmer over medium heat, add the oats and the other ingredients, bring to a simmer and cook for 20 minutes.
2. Divide the mix into bowls and serve for breakfast.

Nutrition info per serving: 393 calories, 6.5g protein, 21.2g carbohydrates, 33.6g fat, 8.6g fiber, 0mg cholesterol, 21mg sodium, 412mg potassium

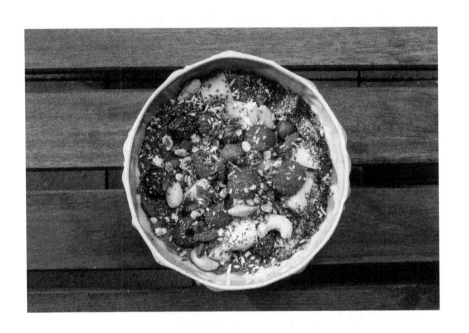

Carrots Hash

Preparation time: 10 minutes

Cooking time: 20 minutes

Servings: 4

Ingredients:

- 2 carrots, peeled and cubed
- 1 tablespoon olive oil
- 1 yellow onion, chopped
- 1 cup low-fat cheddar cheese, shredded
- 8 eggs, whisked
- 1 cup coconut milk
- A pinch of salt and black pepper

Directions:

1. Heat up a pan with the oil over medium heat, add the onion and the carrots, toss and brown for 5 minutes.
2. Add the eggs and the other ingredients, toss, cook for 15 minutes stirring often, divide between plates and serve.

Nutrition info per serving: 431 calories, 20g protein, 9.9g carbohydrates, 35.9g fat, 2.7g fiber,

357mg cholesterol, 330mg sodium, 441mg potassium

Spring Omelet

Preparation time: 10 minutes

Cooking time: 15 minutes

Servings: 4

Ingredients:

- 4 eggs, whisked
- A pinch of black pepper
- ¼ cup low-sodium bacon, chopped
- 1 tablespoon olive oil
- 1 cup red bell peppers, chopped
- 4 spring onions, chopped
- ¾ cup low-fat cheese, shredded

Directions:

1. Heat up a pan with the oil over medium heat, add the spring onions and the bell peppers, toss and cook for 5 minutes.
2. Add the eggs and the other ingredients, toss, spread into the pan, cook for 5 minutes, flip, cook for another 5 minutes, divide between plates and serve.

Nutrition info per serving: 236 calories, 13.9g protein, 4g carbohydrates, 18.8g fat, 0.8g fiber,

205mg cholesterol, 365mg sodium, 178mg potassium

Cheese Frittata

Preparation time: 10 minutes

Cooking time: 20 minutes

Servings: 4

Ingredients:

- A pinch of black pepper
- 4 eggs, whisked
- 2 tablespoons parsley, chopped
- 1 tablespoon low-fat cheese, shredded
- 1 red onion, chopped
- 1 tablespoon olive oil

Directions:

1. Heat up a pan with the oil over medium heat, add the onion and the black pepper, stir and sauté for 5 minutes.
2. Add the eggs mixed with the other ingredients, spread into the pan, introduce in the oven and cook at 360 degrees F for 15 minutes.
3. Divide the frittata between plates and serve.

Nutrition info per serving: 112 calories, 6.3g protein, 3.1g carbohydrates, 8.5g fat, 0.7g fiber, 166mg cholesterol, 75mg sodium, 111mg potassium

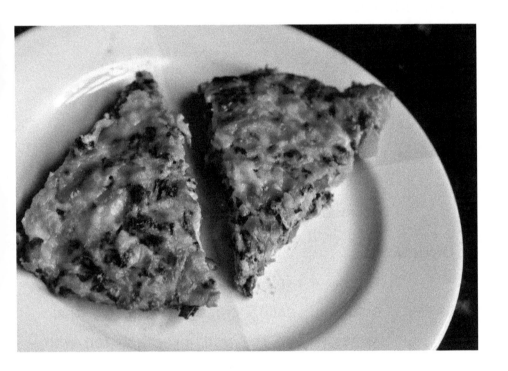

Eggs and Artichokes

Preparation time: 5 minutes

Cooking time: 20 minutes

Servings: 4

Ingredients:

- 4 eggs
- 4 slices low-fat cheddar, shredded
- 1 yellow onion, chopped
- 1 tablespoon avocado oil
- 1 tablespoon cilantro, chopped
- 1 cup canned no-salt-added artichokes, drained and chopped

Directions:

1. Grease 4 ramekins with the oil, divide the onion in each, crack an egg in each ramekin, add the artichokes and top with cilantro and cheddar cheese.
2. Introduce the ramekins in the oven and bake at 380 degrees F for 20 minutes.
3. Serve the baked eggs for breakfast.

Nutrition info per serving: 178 calories, 14.2g protein, 8.4g carbohydrates, 10.9g fat, 2.9g fiber,

184mg cholesterol, 331mg sodium, 261mg potassium

Beans Bake

Preparation time: 10 minutes

Cooking time: 30 minutes

Servings: 8

Ingredients:

- 8 eggs, whisked
- 2 red onions, chopped
- 1 red bell pepper, chopped
- 4 ounces canned black beans, no-salt-added, drained and rinsed
- ½ cup green onions, chopped
- 1 cup low-fat mozzarella cheese, shredded
- Cooking spray

Directions:

1. Grease a baking pan with the cooking spray and spread the black beans, onions, green onions and bell pepper into the pan.
2. Add the eggs mixed with the cheese, introduce in the oven and bake at 380 degrees F for 30 minutes.
3. Divide the mix between plates and serve for breakfast.

Nutrition info per serving: 171 calories, 12.3g protein, 13.7g carbohydrates, 7.8g fat, 3.1g fiber, 175mg cholesterol, 153mg sodium, 365mg potassium

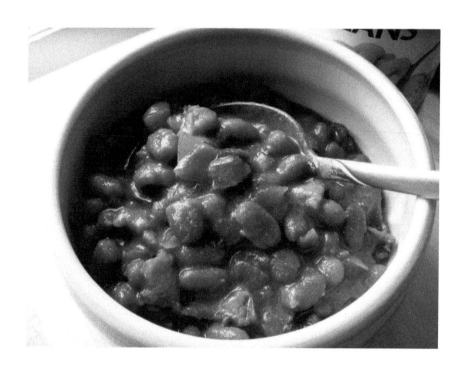

Mozzarella Scramble

Preparation time: 10 minutes

Cooking time: 15 minutes

Servings: 4

Ingredients:

- 3 tablespoons low-fat mozzarella, shredded
- A pinch of black pepper
- 4 eggs, whisked
- 1 red bell pepper, chopped
- 1 teaspoon turmeric powder
- 1 tablespoon olive oil
- 2 shallots, chopped

Directions:

1. Heat up a pan with the oil over medium heat, add the shallots and the bell pepper, stir and sauté for 5 minutes.
2. Add the eggs mixed with the rest of the ingredients, stir, cook for 10 minutes, divide everything between plates and serve.

Nutrition info per serving: 133 calories, 10.2g protein, 5.6g carbohydrates, 8g fat, 1g fiber, 166mg cholesterol, 184mg sodium, 171mg potassium

Cheddar Hash Browns

Preparation time: 10 minutes

Cooking time: 20 minutes

Servings: 4

Ingredients:

- 1 tablespoon olive oil
- 4 eggs, whisked
- 1 cup hash browns
- ½ cup fat-free cheddar cheese, shredded
- 1 small yellow onion, chopped
- A pinch of black pepper
- ½ green bell pepper, chopped
- ½ red bell pepper, chopped
- 1 carrot, chopped
- 1 tablespoon cilantro, chopped

Directions:

1. Heat up a pan with the oil over medium-high heat, add the onion and the hash browns and cook for 5 minutes.
2. Add the bell peppers and the carrots, toss and cook for 5 minutes more.

3. Add the eggs, black pepper and the cheese, stir and cook for another 10 minutes.

4. Add the cilantro, stir, cook for a couple more seconds, divide everything between plates and serve for breakfast.

Nutrition info per serving: 274 calories, 10.8g protein, 19.1g carbohydrates, 17.5g fat, 2.3g fiber, 179mg cholesterol, 295mg sodium, 415mg potassium

Chives Risotto

Preparation time: 10 minutes

Cooking time: 25 minutes

Servings: 4

Ingredients:

- 3 slices bacon, low-sodium, chopped
- 1 tablespoon avocado oil
- 1 cup white rice
- 1 red onion, chopped
- 2 cups low-sodium chicken stock
- 2 tablespoons low-fat parmesan, grated
- 1 tablespoon chives, chopped
- A pinch of black pepper

Directions:

1. Heat up a pan with the oil over medium-high heat, add the onion and the bacon, stir and cook for 5 minutes.
2. Add the rice and the other ingredients, toss, bring to a simmer and cook over medium heat for 20 minutes.
3. Stir the mix, divide into bowls and serve for breakfast.

Nutrition info per serving: 220 calories, 6.4g protein, 39.9g carbohydrates, 3.3g fat, 1.4g fiber, 7mg cholesterol, 219mg sodium, 137mg potassium

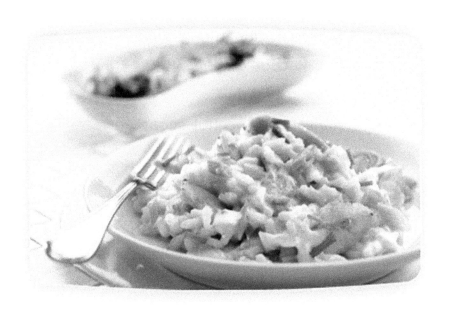

Coconut Quinoa

Preparation time: 5 minutes

Cooking time: 10 minutes

Servings: 4

Ingredients:

- 1 and ½ cups water
- 1 teaspoon cinnamon powder
- 1 and ½ cups quinoa
- 1 cup almond milk
- 1 tablespoon coconut sugar
- ¼ cup pistachios, chopped

Directions:

1. Put the water and the almond milk in a pot, bring to a boil over medium heat, add the quinoa and the other ingredients, whisk, cook for 10 minutes, divide in to bowls, cool down and serve for breakfast.

Nutrition info per serving: 404 calories, 11.1g protein, 48.2g carbohydrates, 19.9g fat, 6.2g fiber, 0mg cholesterol, 32mg sodium, 555mg potassium

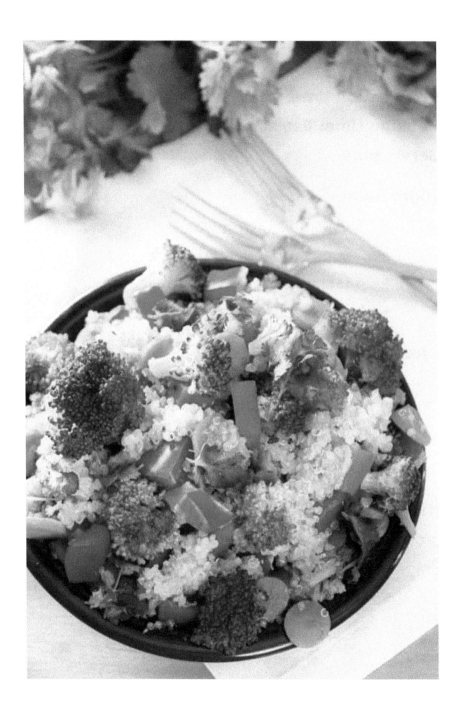

Cherries Bowls

Preparation time: 10 minutes

Cooking time: 0 minutes

Servings: 4

Ingredients:

- 4 cups non-fat yogurt
- 1 cup cherries, pitted and halved
- 4 tablespoons coconut sugar
- ½ teaspoon vanilla extract

Directions:

1. In a bowl, combine the yogurt with the cherries, sugar and vanilla, toss and keep in the fridge for 10 minutes.
2. Divide into bowls and serve f breakfast.

Nutrition info per serving: 205 calories, 14.1g protein, 361.g carbohydrates, 0.5g fat, 0.1g fiber, 5mg cholesterol, 192mg sodium, 645mg potassium

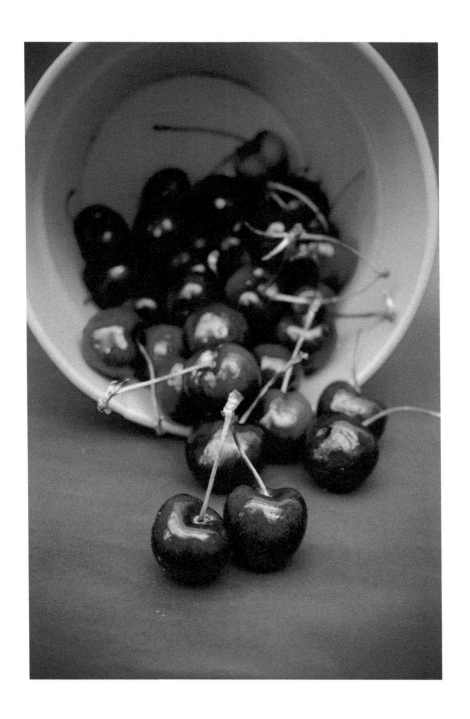

Lightning Source UK Ltd.
Milton Keynes UK
UKHW020815180621
385734UK00005B/58